THE RIGHT WAY TO PHYSICAL HEALTH

SABAT BEATTO

Sidewalk Publisher Inc.
1348 Elder Ave. Bronx, NY 10472

Email: sabeatto@gmail.com

Terms and Conditions

LEGAL NOTICE

The Publisher has strived to be as accurate and complete as possible in the creation of this report, notwithstanding the fact that he does not warrant or represent at any time that the contents within are accurate due to the rapidly changing nature of the Internet.

While all attempts have been made to verify information provided in this publication, the Publisher assumes no responsibility for errors, omissions, or contrary interpretation of the subject matter herein. Any perceived slights of specific persons, peoples, or organizations are unintentional.

In practical advice books, like anything else in life, there are no guarantees of income made. Readers are cautioned to reply on their own judgment about their individual circumstances to act accordingly.

This book is not intended for use as a source of legal, business, accounting or financial advice. All readers are advised to seek services of competent professionals in legal, business, accounting and finance fields.

You are encouraged to print this book for easy reading.

Table Of Contents

Foreword

Chapter 1:
Introduction

Chapter 2:
The Importance Of Maintaining A Strong Body Today And Into The Future

Chapter 3:
Make Sure You Know Your Limitations prior to Taking on an Exercise Regimen

Chapter 4:
Why Stretching Is Important

Chapter 5:
Cardio Training For A Healthy Body

Chapter 6:
Strength Training For A Healthy Body

Chapter 7:
Do You Need A Gym Or Can You Train At Home

Chapter 8:
Outside Activities for Healthy Exercise

Chapter 9:
Exercises You Can Do Anywhere

Chapter 10:
The Benefits Of Learning To Exercise Correctly

Wrapping Up

Foreword

Although being healthy is really based on the unique body constitution of an individual. That is the reason why there is no definite menu for good health. Fortunately, what comes close is the combination regular exercise and the consumption of healthy food. Most of the health programs nowadays talk about coming up with a healthy diet coupled with exercise. Get all the info you need here.

Exercise Your Way To Physical Health
Keeping Your Body Strong With The Right Exercise

Chapter 1:

Over the past years, there has been a growing focus on living longer and looking awesome. All the available medical evidences point to the fact that consistent exercise is the most uncomplicated and pleasing way of maintaining great health.

A massive percentage of the human populace spends most of their days in deskbound jobs and their nights as couch potatoes in front of their television sets. To these people, setting aside some time each day for even the minutest form of exercise may require determination of the highest level. A lot have tried but have gone lukewarm at some point.

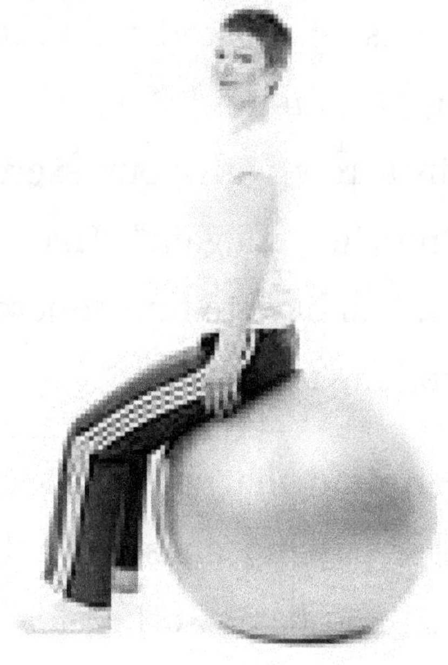

The Basics

One of the essential components of effectively focusing on exercise is to have the proper mindset. You have to keep in mind that keeping fit and looking good is not only for models, actors, and athletes. One can never be too young or too old or too heavy to sign up for a workout plan. There is no denying that constant physical activity is the key to having a healthier, more fit body. Studies also prove that exercise, consistent exercise, is the secret to living a stress-free, contented life.

Regular exercise can enhance an individual's overall well-being. With stress-reducing exercise, chronic illnesses are prevented as well as other heart-related diseases and even premature death.

If you have not exercised for a long time, you have to remember that you need to take things slowly and carefully. Your initial goal is to be able to perform exercises at least three times a week with each exercise session lasting 30 minutes. Make sure that you do not skip more than two days in a row with your exercise program. Do not believe in the saying "no pain, no gain". That may prove to be more harmful than beneficial. You have to remember that pain is the body's way of saying that something is not right.

People have to keep in mind that exercise is requires a lifetime of commitment. It is not a passing phase or a fad. The moment you cease exercising, all that you have worked for will all be for naught. With exercise, patience is crucial. There are no shortcuts, you will not lose lots of poundage in just a few days of workout. The speed of weight loss varies for each individual. A regimen that works well for a friend may not have the same quick and positive effect on you. However, your efforts in exercising will surely be rewarded with good health and active mind.

Health is truly wealth and you have to do what you can to maintain it.

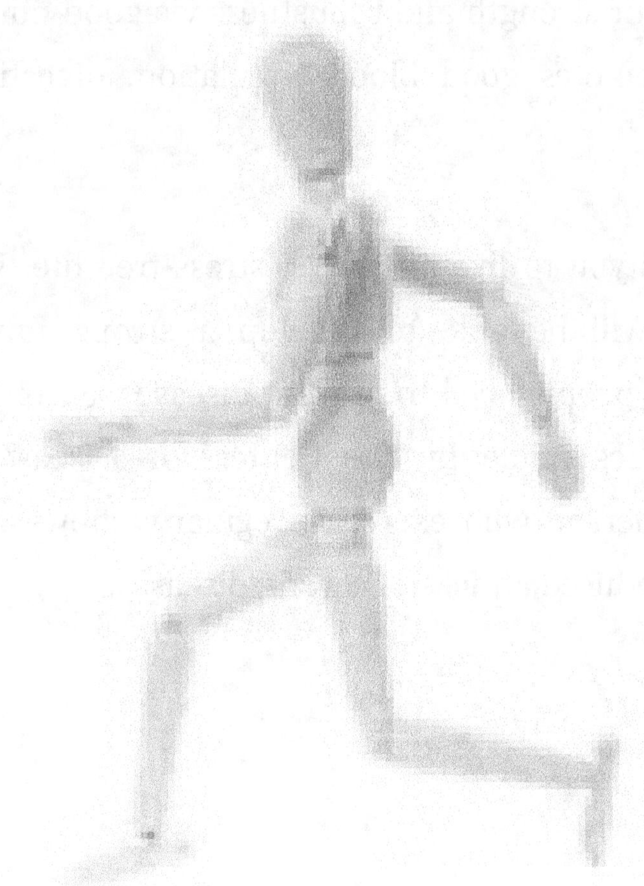

Chapter 2:

The Importance Of Maintaining A Strong Body Today And Into The Future

Having a healthy body prepares the stage for your everyday well-being. It also has a direct impact on how fast and fine you will age. Maintaining your strength and robustness via good nutrition and lots of exercise promotes good blood circulation, digestion, and bone strength.

Exercise allows you to live an active, stress-free life. With plenty of exercise, you will be able to develop a strong immune system, something that people need to prevent diseases, chronic and serious. Based on studies made by the Center for Disease Control and Prevention, a person who exercises regularly shows greater mental alertness and reduced attacks of certain diseases.

Why It's Important

When your metabolism is working at its peak, you are able to burn more calories which your body uses for energy. This would also result in lesser aches and pains. The body needs lots of vitamins, dietary fiber, minerals, carbohydrates, and fatty acids in order to allow all body processes to function properly. Regular night bed rest is also necessary.

When you sleep, the body goes into work and repairs damaged cells. Deficiency in sleep, good nutrition, and exercise can deny the body of essential elements that will result in fatigue and stress.

 The national Sleep Foundation says that ample sleep makes you less vulnerable to colds and flu. Getting enough exercise and the right kind of food can leave a person physically and mentally sharp. Constant workouts prepare the different parts of the body like the muscles, heart, lungs, and bones for the demands of daily life.

When the body reaches a healthy level and stays on that plateau, it would be able to withstand extraordinary stress and it would les likely give in to simple infections and other common diseases. When you do regular exercise such as aerobics, you effectively toughen your muscles and bones and this helps you avoid sprains, bone fractures, and even pulled muscles.

When you are fit, you can move more. Movement promotes calorie burning and this will eventually aid you in maintaining your weight. Half an hour of exercise each day will balance your calorie intake, this according to the American Heart Association.

Partner exercise with foods that are rich in fiber and low in fat can greatly help you control your weight. High fiber nutrition also encourages a healthy cardiovascular system.

Maintaining the right body weight reduces the risk of developing cardiovascular diseases as well as other forms of cancer and type 2 diabetes. These diseases do not progress in a short period of time, they develop through the years, and that is the reason why keeping your body healthy and fit is your best shot at preventing these types of diseases.

A healthy body maintained by exercise is your passport to a more meaningful and longer life.

Chapter 3:

Make Sure You Know Your Limitations prior to Taking on an Exercise Regimen

Making the decision to integrate regular exercise into your daily life can be a life-changing choice for you. It is definitely a smart move to leave lethargy behind and switch into a healthier, more active lifestyle instead of bumming in front of the boob tube while eating chips.

Nevertheless, exercise can be precarious especially for people who have specific health issues and those who have not done any strenuous physical activity for a long time.

Obese people are also advised to consult health specialists before embarking on an exercise regimen. Immediately going on board a demanding type of workout can lead to serious body injury. It is important to be familiar with the steps.

Your Limits

Knowing Your Limitations

If you have not heard of PAR-Q, it is the standard used to gauge fitness safety. This tool is used by health clubs, physical trainers, and even doctors all over the world. The name is short for Physical Activity Readiness Questionnaire and it is usually composed of 5 to 7 questions that can help a person determine if there are any health concerns that need to be addressed before undergoing an exercise program. These questions are answerable by yes or no. Here are some of the questions:

- Has your doctor prescribed you with drugs for blood pressure control or any hart condition?
- Are you suffering from any joint or bone problem which could be made worse if you undergo any strenuous physical activity?
- Have you ever lost balance because you felt dizzy? Do you occasionally lose consciousness?
- Have you experienced chest pains in the past even if you are not performing any physical activity? Do you feel pain in your chest when you perform physical activity?
- Has your doctor diagnosed you as having a heart condition? Has your doctor ordered you to refrain from doing any physical activity that he did not recommend?

If your answer is yes to any of these questions, it is best to consult your doctor and get cleared before you start with any type of workout.

Aside from this, here are other high risk conditions that require a go-signal from the doctor before the individual begins exercising:

- Being 20 pounds overweight
- Chain smoker
- Suffering from arthritis
- Having high blood pressure
- Diabetes
- Other chronic medical conditions

This does not mean that you cannot do exercise if you are hypertensive or diabetic. In fact, exercising is more often than not an essential part of treatment for these types of conditions. However, you may have limitations and your doctor is the best person to help you with these special concerns.

The rule in exercise is to always begin slowly until you have built enough intensity to level up your workouts. Gradual is the name of the game, not abrupt. Doing a hundred sit ups on your first day of exercise (although it is doubtful if you can do it) is a prescription to serious health issues.

Chapter 4:

Why Stretching Is Important

As we mature, our muscles constrict and tighten. This makes the range of motion in our joints curtailed and minimized. This state can negatively affect our active lifestyles and even hold back every day, normal motion. Household tasks that used to be simple, like for instance bowing or even reaching for a can off of the top of the fridge, now become tremendously complicated.

A regular stretching program can help lengthen your muscles and make daily living activities easier.

Almost everyone can learn to stretch, regardless of age or flexibility. Stretching should actually be a part of a person's daily habits. This means that we have to stretch whether we want to exercise or not. There are simple stretches you can do while doing a lot of things. You can even do stretches while in front of the TV, after a long night's sleep, or before going to bed. You have to do stretches in between sets If you are doing strength training exercises. Stretching makes you feel good and it prepares you for the workout ahead.

Stretching

Stretching does not require a lot of time. Despite this, stretching can really help you achieve amazing results with your workouts. Here are some of the many benefits that you get from regular stretching:

- Increased blood circulation to the different parts of the body
- Boosted energy levels
- Less muscle tension
- Increased flexibility and movement in the joints
- Improved muscular synchronization

Stretching offers a lot of advantages to people of different ages. As already mentioned, one of the benefits of stretching is the increase of one's range of motion,. This means your joints and limbs can budge and move about further before an injury happens. Post-exercise stretching can also help in workout recuperation, reduce muscle discomfort, and make certain that your muscles and tendons are in good working order.

The more hardened and toned your muscles and tendons are, the better they can cope with the rigors of sport and exercise. This also means that your chances of becoming injured are less compared to if you did not perform stretching.

Stretching, when you actually think of it, is natural to all of us. You have most likely noticed that if you have been sitting in a particular position for a long time, you stretch automatically even without thinking. Stretching alleviates tension and it makes you feel good.

Aside from that amazingly good feeling after a stretch, your muscle and bones become more limber. You have to take care of your muscles and they will definitely return the favor.

Work and other non-exercise activities can cause tension. Tension can lead to pains in the muscles. Stretching helps relax your muscles, it aids in the prevention of muscle cramps. Yoga practitioners have used stretching as a meditation technique to help focus the mind. This helps you take your mind off other stressful things relieving you of anxiety and pressure. Post workout stretching will definitely help you improve your flexibility and reduce the chances of injury.

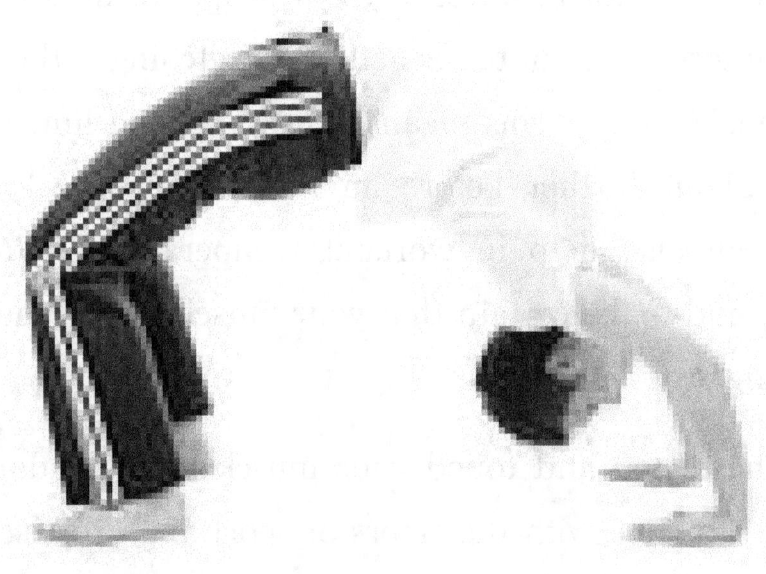

Chapter 5:

Cardio training is any form of training that amplifies the work of the lungs and the heart. Some of the most common forms of cardio training include walking, jogging, running, and biking. Other forms of cardio training include swimming, cross training, and rowing.

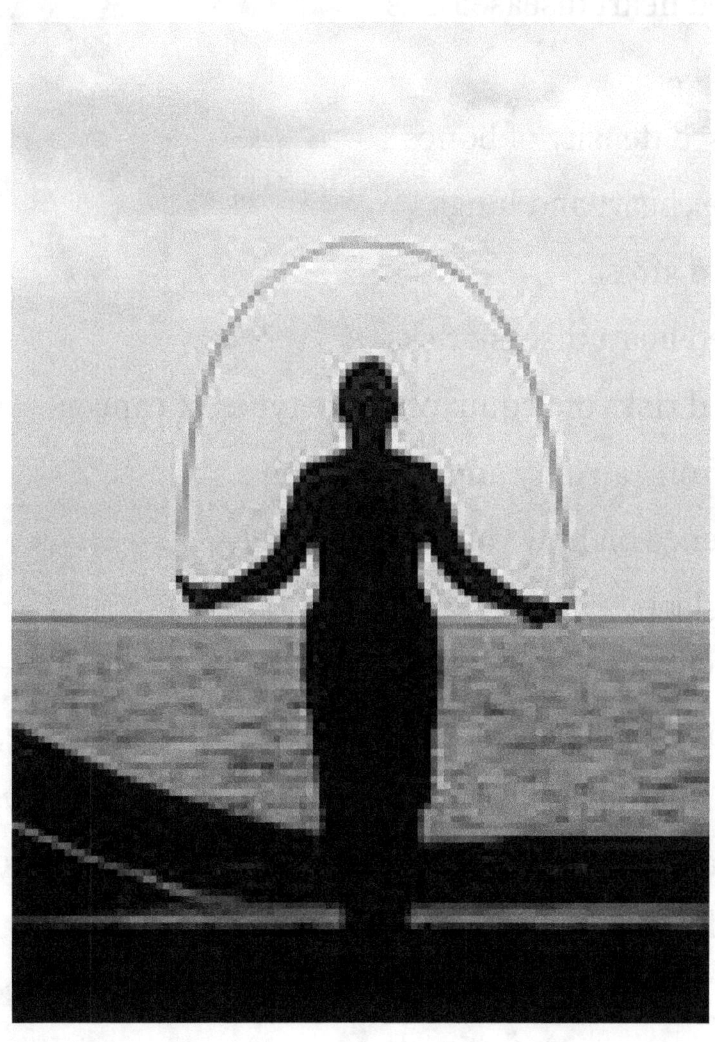

Cardio

The benefits of cardio training are limitless and they include:

- Improved muscle mass
- Less risk of osteoporosis
- Enhanced heart function
- Enhanced blood cholesterol and triglyceride levels
- Reduced heart disease risks
- Weight loss
- Increased density of bones
- Stronger heart and lungs
- Reduced stress
- Reduced heart disease risks
- Reduced risks of acquiring some types of cancer
- Relief from anxiety and depression
- Confidence on how you look and feel
- Better sleep

According to the American College of Sports Medicine, an average adult should spend at least 30 minutes of moderate physical activity at least 4 days a week. There is no denying it, cardio training is essential in the development of a healthy body.

Our Bodies Have been Designed To Move

If you have a deskbound job, you can just imagine how your body feels towards the end of each working day. Have you noticed that you have tight muscles, a painful back, and you feel totally worn out even though you really have not done anything remotely similar to a total workout? Your shoulders may be burning from tension and your head hurts from gazing at the computer screen for the longest time. Afterwards, imagine how the body feels after a real workout. Your muscles become warm and lithe, the blood is freely flowing through your entire body delivering much needed oxygen and energy. You feel keyed up, positive and even proud of yourself. The feeling is entirely different. Our bodies are designed for motion--not stay at one place and sit around the whole day.

Cardio Results in Better Life Quality

Today, appearance is significant. People have become really preoccupied with how they look that at some point, they do not really care how they feel. If you lf take a second look at the benefits mentioned, all of them point to the direction of feeling good not only now but in the future as well.

Cardio training promotes movement and this increase blood flow. Cardio training reinforces the heart and lungs and trains the heart to work more efficiently. When you perform cardio training, you also set a good example for your kids and this could spell a better future for them.

Performing cardiovascular workouts also positively modifies the hormonal features of your body significantly. It releases 'feel good' hormones that will help relieve signs of despair and exhaustion as well as releasing appetite decreasing hormones. In the end, cardio exercises aids in healthy gradual weight loss. This is great for people not only for people who are overweight but for those who have health issues like diabetes and hypertension, conditions that are worsened by excess body fat.

Chapter 6:
Strength Training For A Healthy Body

Strength training is the type of work out that employs resistance to make stronger and shape up the skeletal and muscular system of the body, enhancing muscle tone and stamina. Strength training is synonymous to other exercise terms such as weightlifting and resistance training.

Strength

The Advantages of Strength Training

Physically, the benefits of steady strength training include a boost in muscle size and tone, increased muscular power, and amplification in bone, tendon, and sinew strength. Strength training has can also develop one's psychological status by increasing confidence and self-esteem.

Here are other worthy benefits of strength training:

• Energy Boost: additional endurance, control and strength which results into more energy
• Better digestion and purging processes. Your body is designed to be active in many ways
• Superior cerebral ability and output. Strength training provides an interval needed by the human brain from the constant thinking jobs which is so ordinary in this modern world.
• Improved sleep: Strength training develops a better sleeping pattern for you.
• Weight loss: with strength training, the muscle burns more calories than fats because of improved metabolism.
• Tougher bones: increased bone mineral density resulting from loads placed on the bones during the strength training

• Depression control: While exercising, the brain sends out endorphins resulting in a happy state of mind during and after exercise
• Reduced stress
• Protection from heart disease: reduced blood pressure and weight loss
• Improved self-confidence and self-perception
• Body fat percentage reduction
• Lean tissue increase
• Strength increases
• Lung function improves
• Bone mineral density increases

Strength training will definitely aid in the increase of mental and physical stamina to help you better tolerate the stresses of life at work and at home. Another one of the many benefits of a good strength training program is its effect on our appearance. A great looking body has a direct correlation to an individual's self-esteem and his level of confidence.

Strength Training Can Slow Down Aging

Strength training is essential in thwarting muscle loss that usually accompanies the aging process. A common false impression is that as we reach grow old, it is normal to stop being active and to begin using canes and wheelchairs. Many think that we have no choice.

The truth is there is completely no reason why all of us can't be bodily, psychologically, and socially active living a healthy life even when we have already matured. The reason why many elderly people have become slower and fatter is simply because over the years, their muscles have wasted away without strength training. This has resulted in the decrease of their body's physical performance and metabolism which is the reason why they have become less efficient.

The body needs consistent strength training in order to slow down muscle and bone weakness. Constant physical movement prepares the body for the rougher road ahead. You will eventually notice that mature people who have had ample physical activity in their youth are still capable of doing a lot things without supervision when they get old.

Chapter 7:

Do You Need A Gym Or Can You Train At Home

Exercising is a smart move, especially if you want to lose weight and improve your overall health. You can perform your exercises at home or in gyms. But the question is, which is more effective, training at home or in a gym? To answer this question, let us take a look at the advantages and disadvantages of both options.

At Home?

What are the benefits to working out at home?

- At home, you can enjoy your privacy. You don't have to sweat it out in full view of a group of strangers.
- You can work out any time you like. You don't have wait until the gym opens and hurry out when it is about to close for the day.
- You don't have to go outdoors especially when the weather is bad to get to the gym.
- You can tailor your home gym to meet your specific fitness needs.
- A home gym is usually less expensive than a gym membership.
- You can make no excuse not to be able to exercise because the gym is right where you are – at home.

Before you decide whether a home gym is right for you, take a look at the following factors:

- Your fitness needs.
- The type of workout that you want.
- Your budget.
- The amount of space you are willing to provide for your home gym equipment.

When you have finally decided that a home gym is the best for you, you will need to carefully pick the best home gym equipment. Several home gym gadgets let you perform several types of exercises on one piece of equipment. This is suitable for people who have limited spaces in their homes. It is also affordable for the average person.

One negative aspect of a home gym is that you do not have access to workout professionals who can help you learn to use the equipment and develop an exercise routine that is best for you.

However, there are a couple of ways you can deal with that. Exercise equipment that you purchase frequently comes with instructional videos. You can watch the video thoroughly. Sales representatives are also trained and they can help you learn to use the equipment. You can also hire a personal trainer for a session or two just to help you get started on your exercise routine.

The Gym

Even though the home gym is the runaway winner when it comes to cost, gym memberships come with several perks that may not be present at home. Some gyms have fitness classes and you have to agree, it is very encouraging to exercise more when you are with peers. Other gyms have spa services and that would be very difficult to duplicate at home. You can even have massage therapy in membership gyms. First class gyms come with complete exercise facilities, something that you would not be able to fit at home.

At the end of the day, it is up to you to decide whether you would go for the home gym or the membership gym, but whatever your pick is, it is a great thing you decided to stretch those muscles.

Chapter 8:

Outside Activities for Healthy Exercise

Exercise needs to be fun in order for you to keep your focus while doing it. Outdoor activities make staying healthy and staying in shape more interesting. Here are some activities that you can also include in your routine that takes boredom from and puts in the fun in exercise.

Get Outside

Go Swimming

Swimming is a popular outdoor activity that stimulates all the muscles in your body. If you have easy access to a pool, go and take the plunge. Swimming can be fun and at the same time, it helps tone your body muscles. Exercising on a treadmill can be a bore most of the time but with swimming, you can cool off, enjoy, and get in shape. You will not even notice how many hours you have spent swimming when you do so.

Doggy Playtime

If you have a dog, it would be the perfect opportunity to have an exercise buddy. When you have a dog, you can exercise by walking or jogging with him. What is great about exercising with your dog, especially if you are a dog lover, is that you won't mind how long it would take for you to walk or jog because you are with your canine best friend. Other than walking, you can also play fetch with your dog or play roughhouse with him. It may not seem strenuous as going on a treadmill for hours, but this type of exercise can be a great workout that benefits both you and your dog.

Go Hiking

Why spend hours and hours on a treadmill just to work on your leg muscles when you can do something more fun like hiking along a nature trail. Hiking works greatly on your leg muscles and you will be more interested when you get to see different things along your journey. You can someone to go with you to make it more exciting. Of course, you can also bring along a camera just in case you come across something remarkably interesting.

Cycling

Cycling is a great cardiovascular exercise that you can enjoy especially when you do it around your community. Some would even opt to cycle to different distances not only as their workout routine but as a way to enjoy different sights. Work those quadriceps while enjoying scenic views when you go cycling.

Go Kayaking

If you aim to work on the muscles of your upper body, go kayaking. This is an ultimate outdoor sport that combines fun, excitement, and workout. When you go kayaking, it is not just about working on your arms; in fact, you will tire easily when you put so much effort on the arms. Instead, work your whole upper body as you row the paddle. Of course, if you want kayaking to be part of your outdoor exercise routine, you need to know different paddling techniques and things to do in case problems arise while on the water. Kayaking targets the muscles on the center of the body, the stomach and back.

These are simply some of the outdoor activities that you can do to put a fun meaning to exercise. Outdoor exercises are ideal if you have all the time to perform them.

Chapter 9:
Exercises You Can Do Anywhere

When you have a hectic daily schedule, it would be hard to find time for exercise especially when there are tons of things to worry about such as packing everyone's lunch, sending the kids to school, work, picking them up from school, cooking dinner, and the list would go on. Exercise should be part of a your daily living especially if you have a busy schedule as it can energize the body and handle stress that can be a cause for obesity.

When you can't find time to do some outdoor exercises, or get on the treadmill for hours for cardio exercises, there are different exercises that you can do just about anytime and anywhere – and this time, no more excuses. Amidst your busy schedule, you can insert a time slot for exercise because there are activities that you can do any place that you think is convenient for you. Keep in mind that you should always start with a warm-up and end with a cool-down exercise.

Do It Anywhere

Pushups

Anyone is familiar with the usual position when performing a pushup. You can modify the boring pushup workout a bit and give variety to it. Try to work more on your chest and shoulder by doing pushups with the hands positioned wider than your shoulders. Halfway pushups can also intensify this type of workout.

Crunches

Doing your crunches correctly can result to a perfectly-toned abs. On the other hand, doing it the wrong way can bring pain to your neck and back. Use correct techniques when doing crunches to help avoid physical injury.

Tricep Dips

Place yourself on the edge of a bench and put your hands next to the thighs. Lift your body outwards to the front of your chair, bending your knees and keeping your feet flat on the ground. Next, you will lower yourself allowing the elbows to bend to not more than 90 degrees, and then push your body back up. This type of exercise is not suitable when you have shoulder or wrist problems.

Squats

Squats are simple exercises that can be done anywhere. With proper techniques, you can have a satisfying workout. Start the squatting exercises by lowering your body by a foot. Gradually take deeper squats during the entire duration of exercise when your muscles have become accustomed to the activity. If you aim to have a more intense workout with squats, hold two sand-filled 2-liter bottles on each hand while you perform this exercise.

There will always be time for exercise. No matter how busy your schedule is, always make little time to do some exercise to keep your body in good shape so you can function better in your daily activities. Remember that you should take things slow at first and know the capabilities of your body. It is good if you feel soreness in your body but if body pains are intense, your body is signaling you to stop. Give these simple exercises a try and feel the difference of being healthy.

Chapter 10:

Some would think that performing exercise can only lead to injury. Undeniably true, exercise when performed the wrong way can harm the body. Before engaging in any sport or activity it is best to learn the proper way of doing it. Although for most people, they only think of starting and finishing an exercise. Unknowingly, when in a wrong posture or stance even in just one move, they already have caused teardown or strained their muscles. Proper body position is one technique to refrain from causing damage to your body.

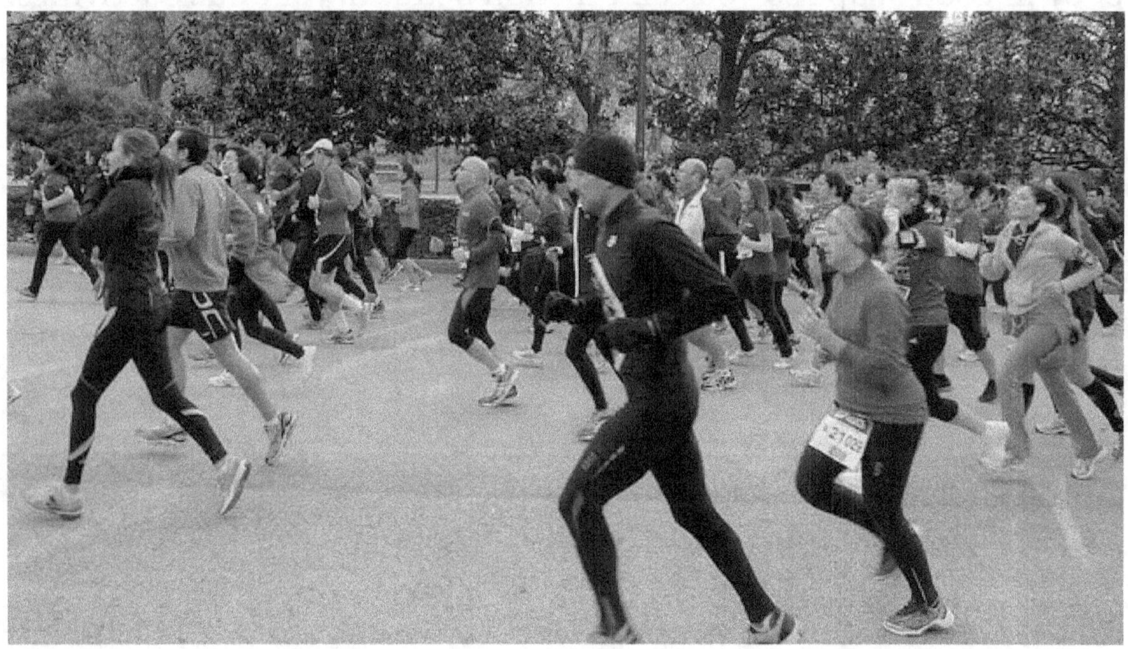

Do it Right

When doing exercise, the body will compensate to maintain balance by increasing muscle strength. The application of biomechanics in every exercise will certainly help not only an athlete but anyone trying to rebuild an injured muscle. The more knowledgeable you are with what exercises to perform, the lesser effort you need to exert to attain your goal.

Always consider the right exercise fit for a specific muscle. Any alteration or movement is critical to the body. The human body always tries to balance whatever changes it feels. Shifting from one position to another must be done properly if you want to stay mobile for a longer time. Keep in mind that some movements are not correct even if it feels good. It is important to keep track on how a specific exercise should be done and not to base only on how it feels like.

If you are new to the world of exercise, prepare your mind and emotion. Never get dismayed right away if you feel that you are not doing the proper way of exercising. Do not set the bar too high but see to it that you engage yourself in doing the exercises well. It always takes time and patience to see results.

It is good to learn slowly and progress the type of exercise once you have mastered one. Proper exercise will enable an individual to attain cardiovascular fitness, good flexibility and excellent muscle strength. Thus, there are reduced chances of muscle or physical injuries even to the most brittle part of the body. Gradual movement and muscle strengthening regimen will help you maximize and enjoy the benefits of exercise. You can start with simple forward reach to better you hamstrings. Perform some forward press to improve your chest and some triceps kickback for your triceps strength.

You might have the notion that you can only learn these proper exercising techniques when you enroll in a gym class. Well not at all, all you need to have is your body and a strong determination. But only if you can, add a simple accessory such as a cheap balance ball to assist you in your moves.

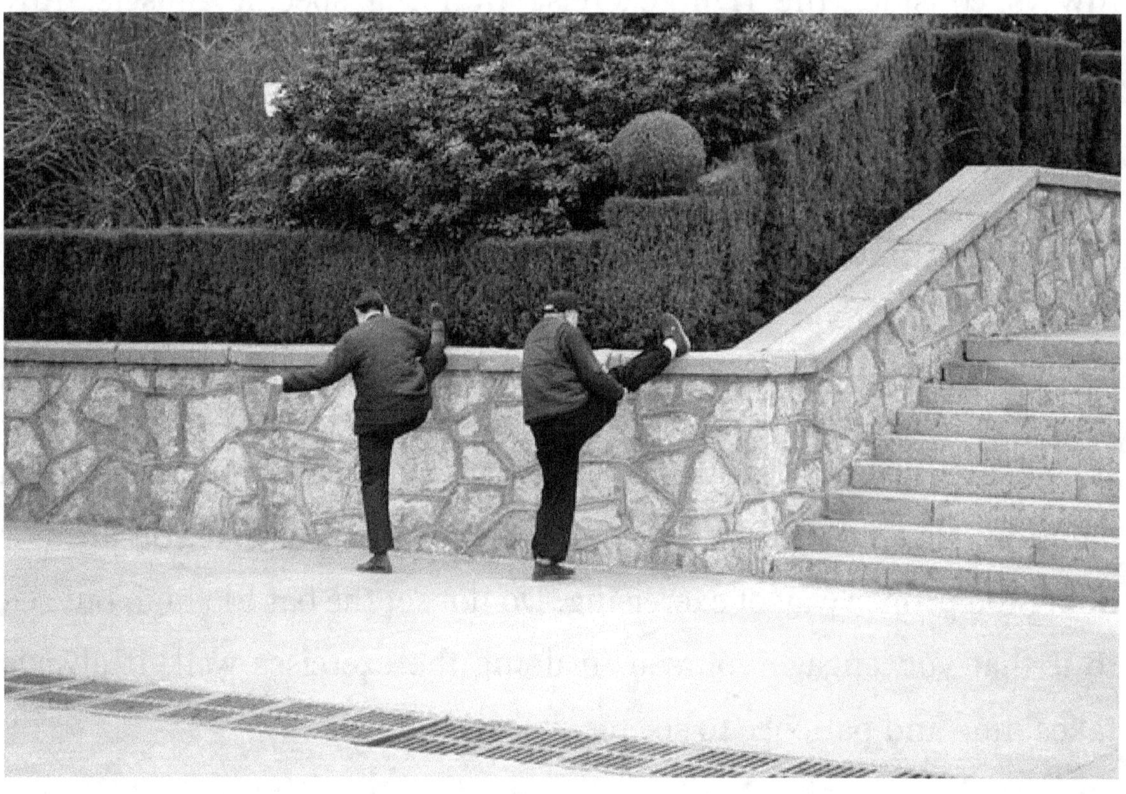

Wrapping Up

Exercise plays a vital role for everyone. It helps improve the body's muscle mass and most of all it helps a person feel good about himself. Exercise does not only help you lose weight but it also serves as a relaxing activity after a stressful day's work. Doing body workout enhances the release of endorphins or happy hormones in the body. This type of hormones improves the well-being of a person. Increased ability to concentrate and higher energy throughout the day are also an advantage when doing exercise.

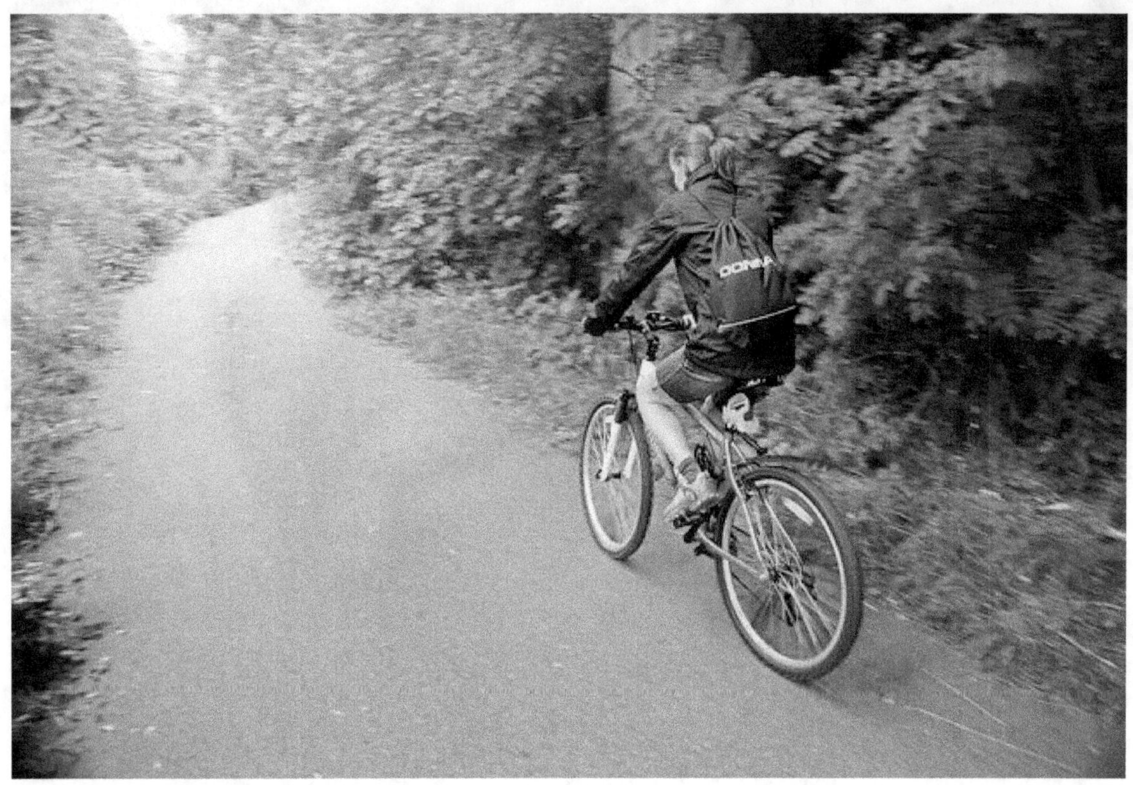

TAKE A NOTE